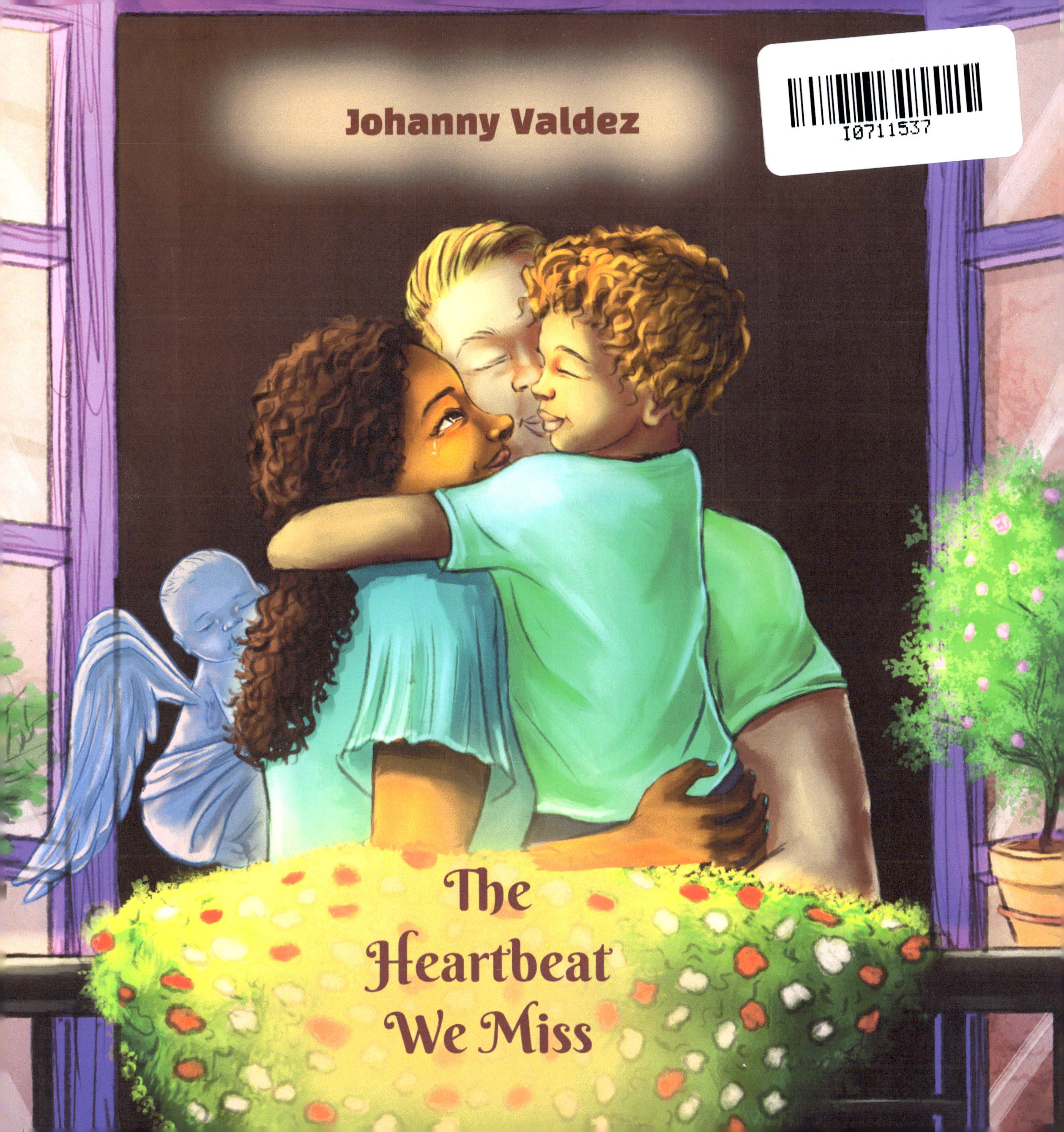

Johanny Valdez
The
Heartbeat
We Miss

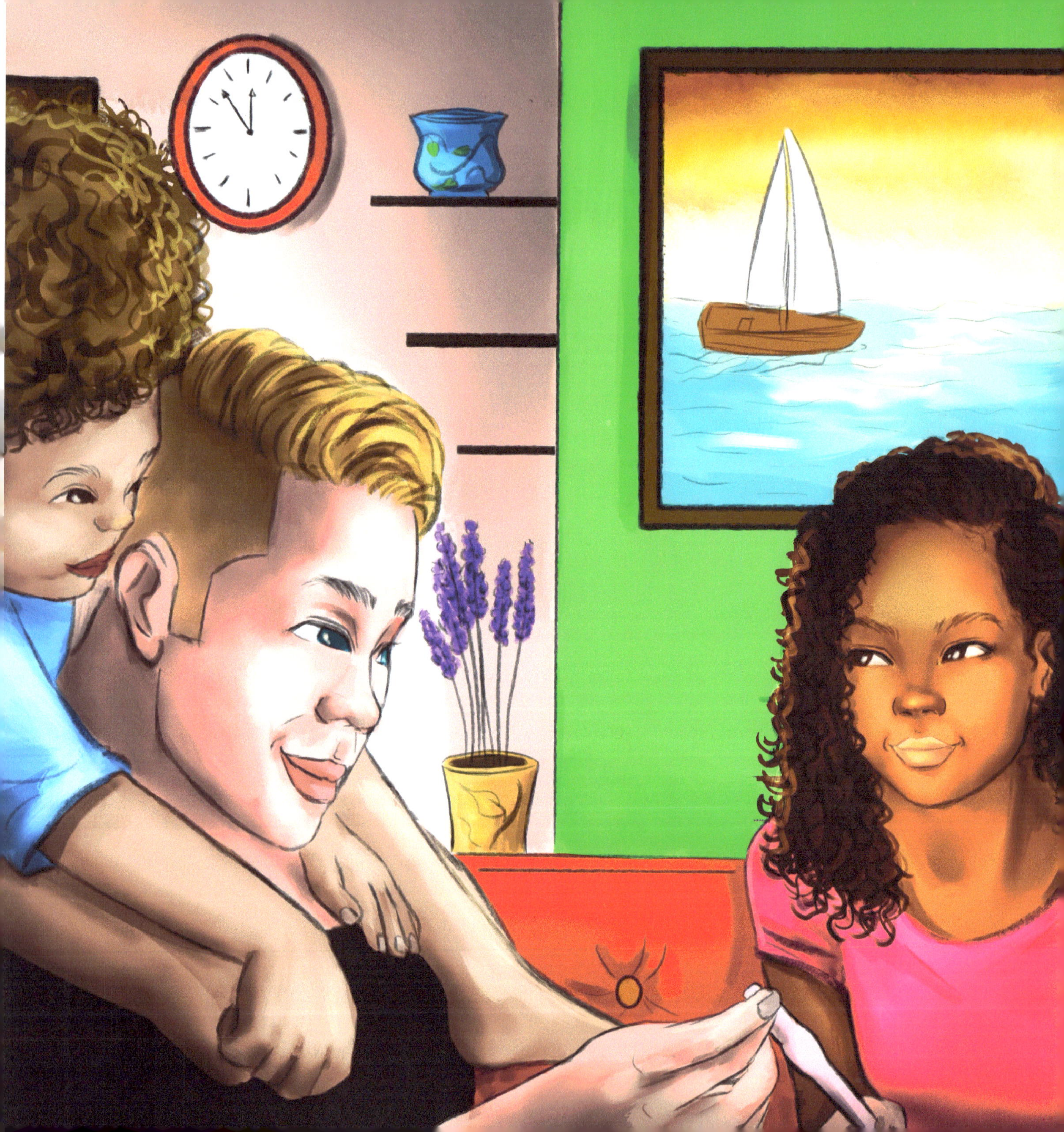

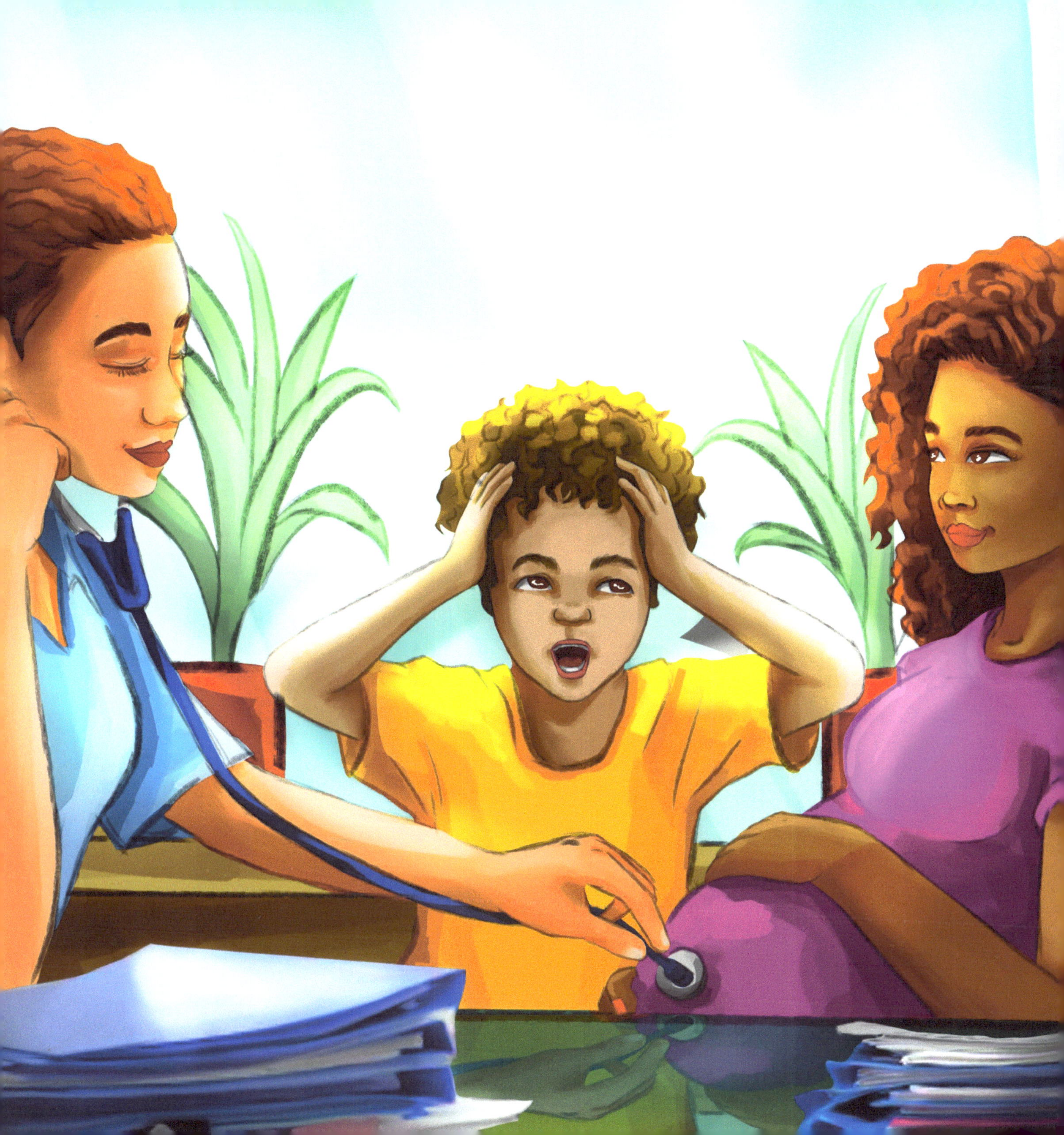

We're all feeling very happy
The family is about to grow
Because a new family member
Is ready to be born

We can hear the baby's heartbeat
It is beating very fast
Right inside of mummy's belly
How amazing is all that!

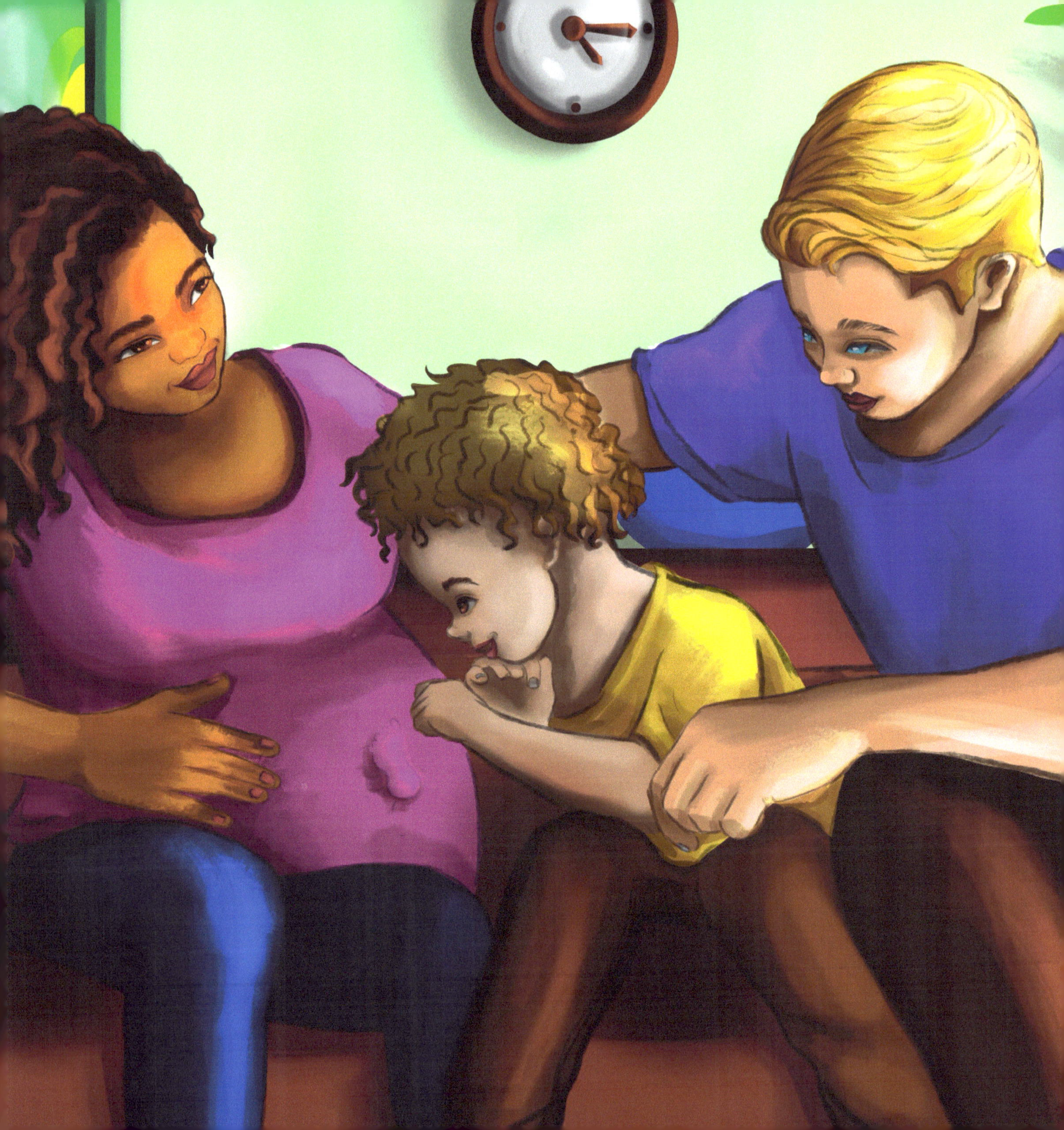

We can see the baby kicking
It is very fun to see
We are jumping with emotion
Mummy, can I blow baby a kiss?

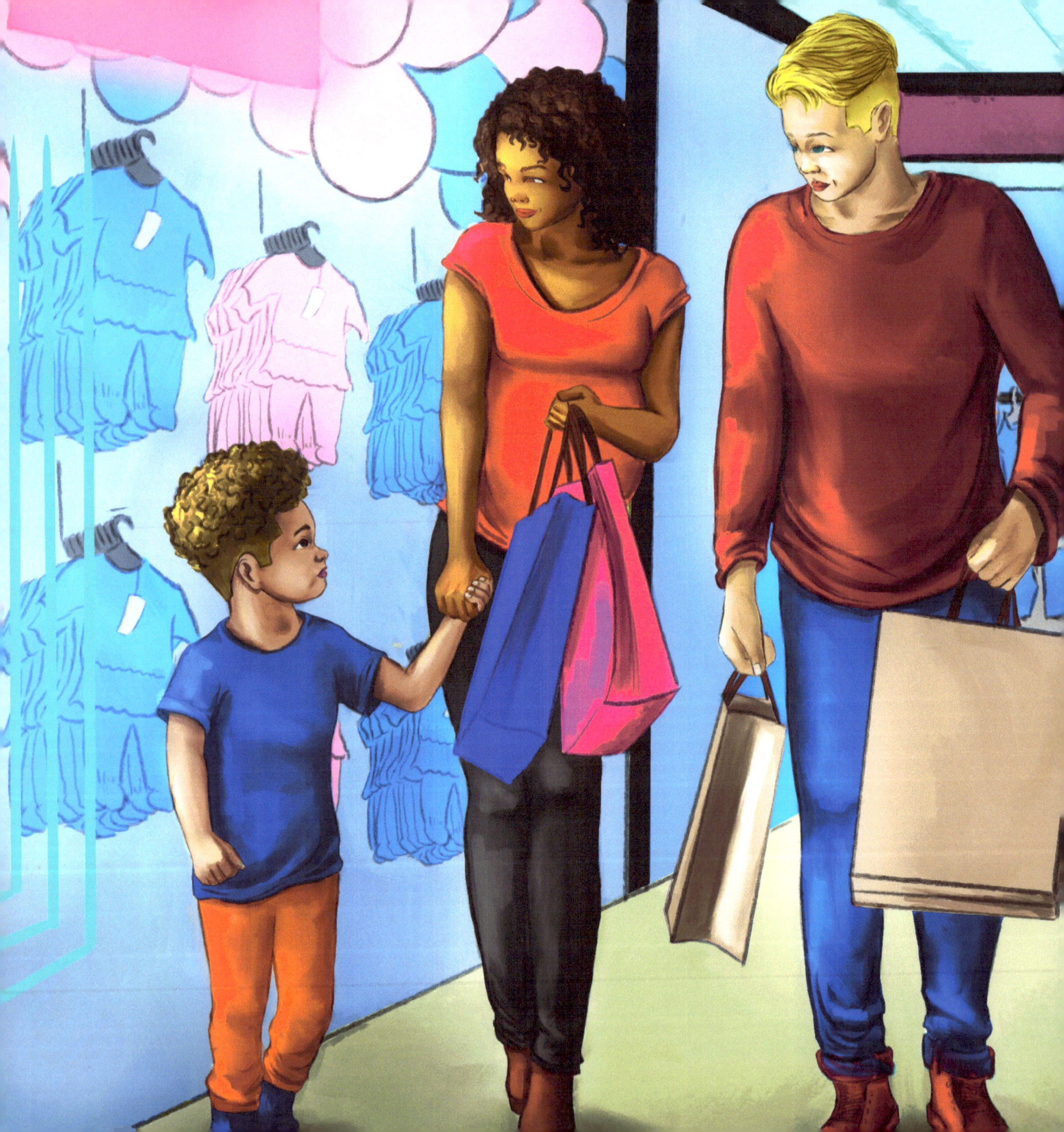

We went shopping for the baby
New clothes and a new crib
We can't wait to dress the baby
And to show him all his things!

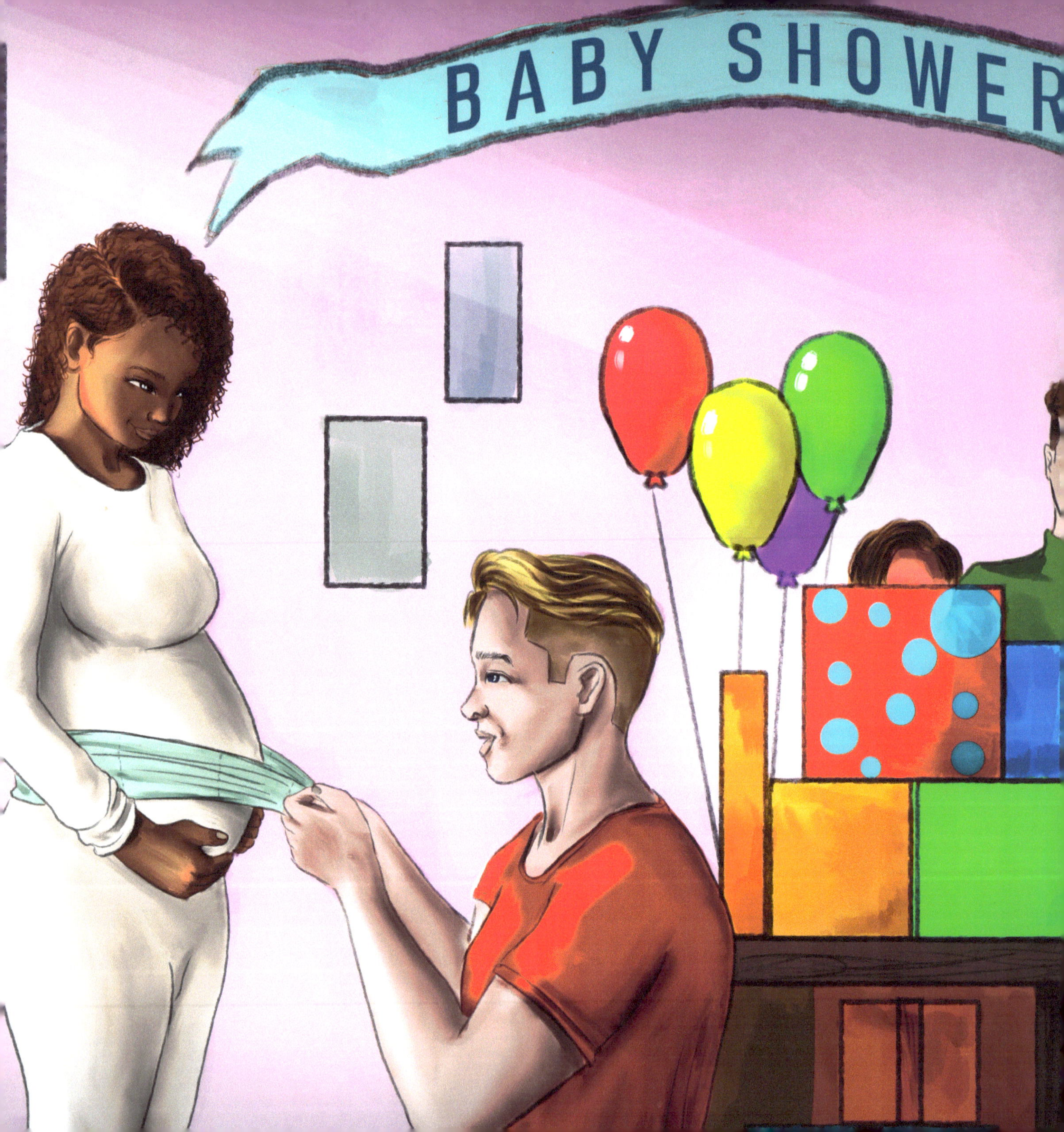
BABY SHOWER

How jolly is the baby shower
Everyone's having so much fun
There is food and many gifts
And good wishes for the mum

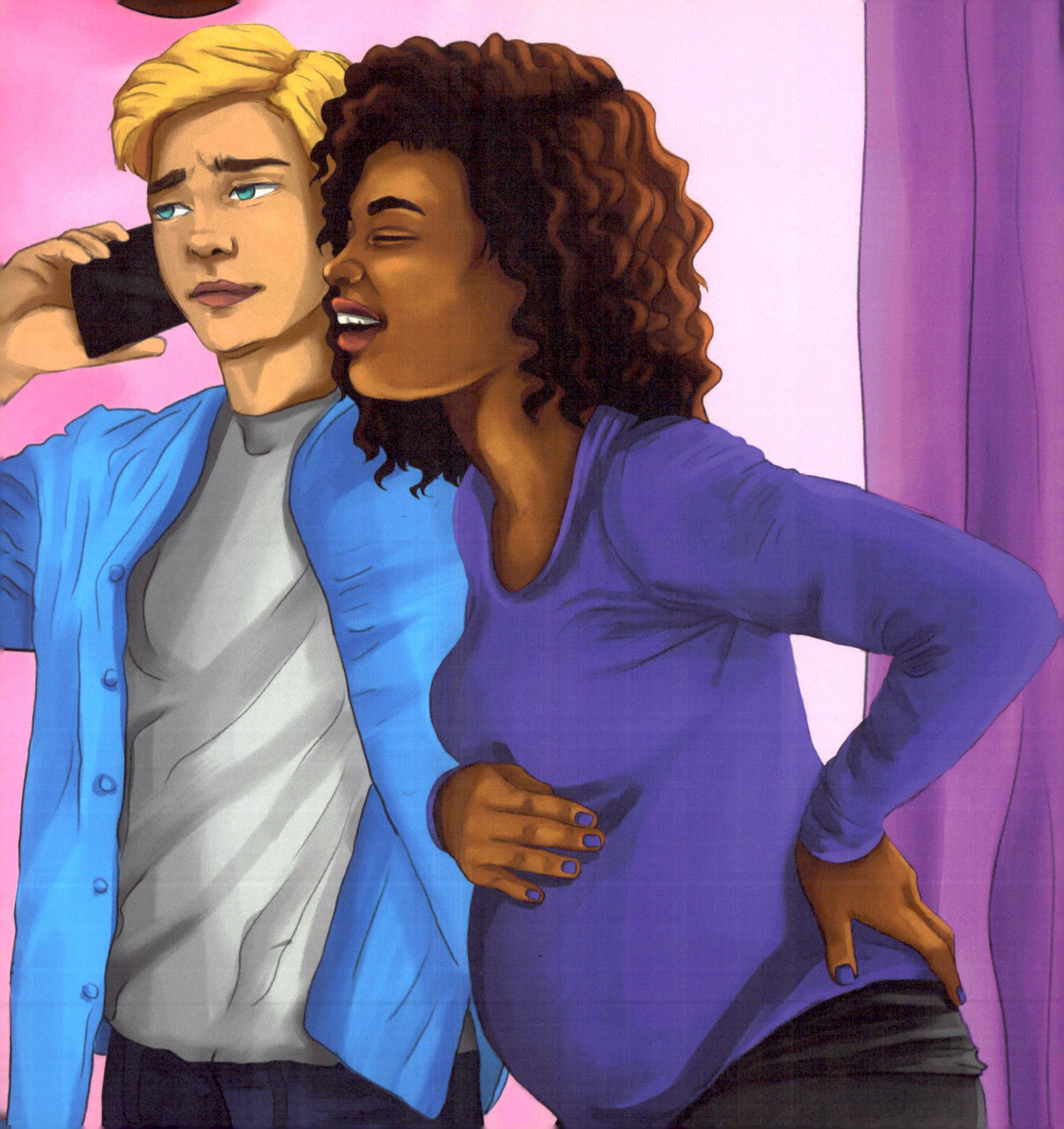

Something strange is going on
Baby seems a bit too quiet
Mum and dad will call the doctor
And we'll go to get an answer

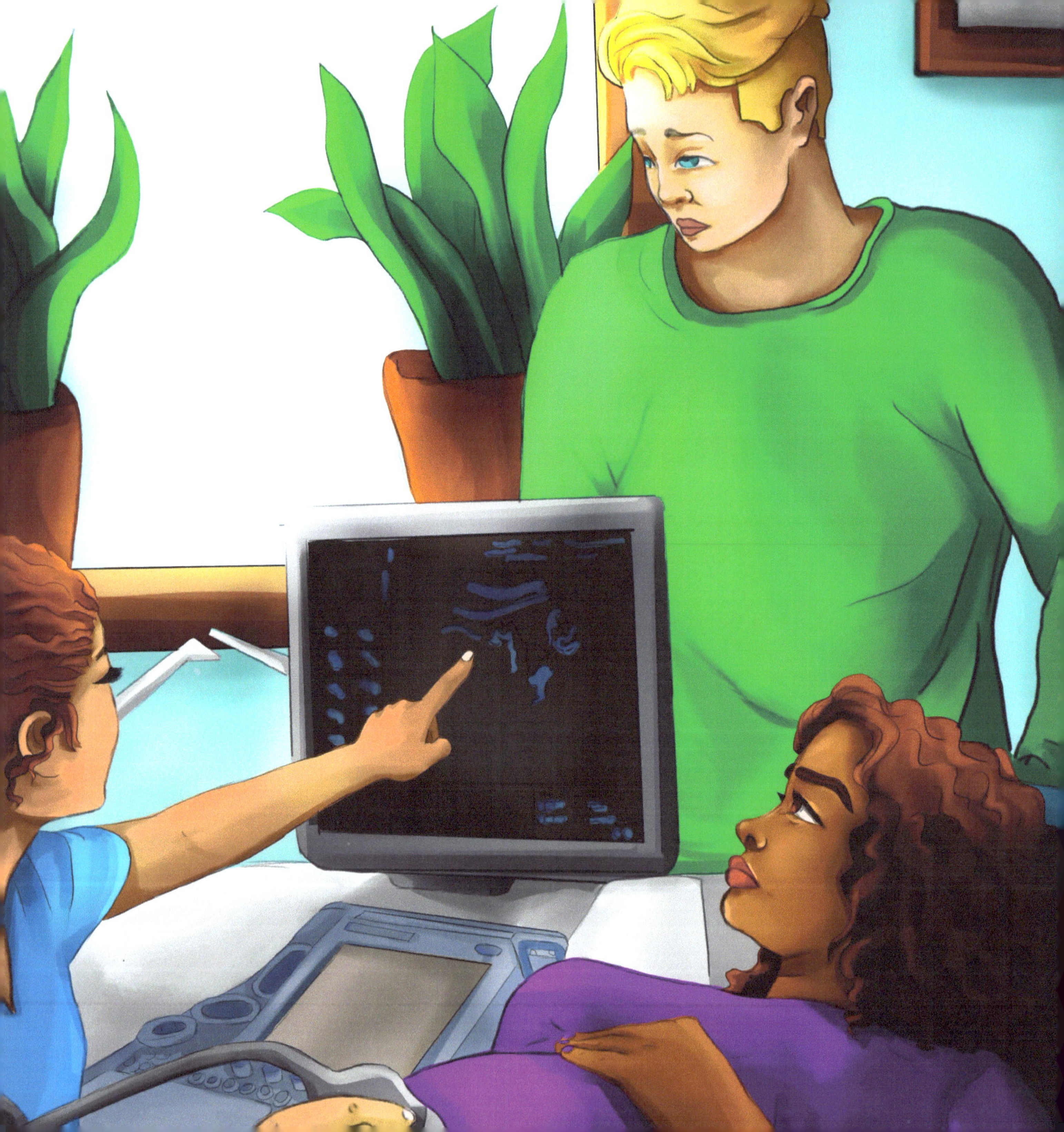

The heartbeat of the baby
We cannot hear this time
We don't understand what happened
Mum and dad look sad with fear

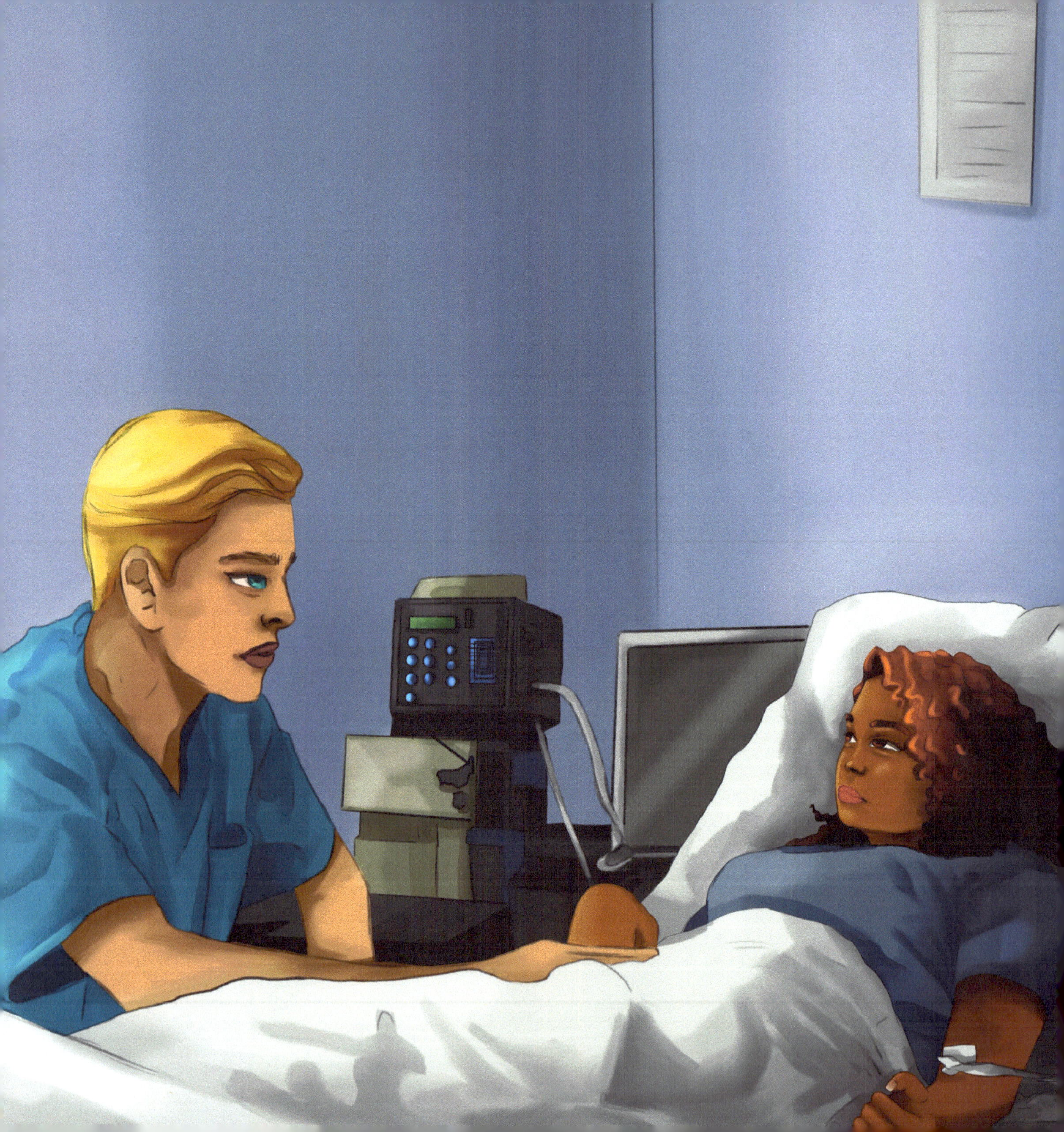

Mum is healing from a surgery
I'm not sure what that was about
Her belly looks so much smaller
There is no baby, we figure out

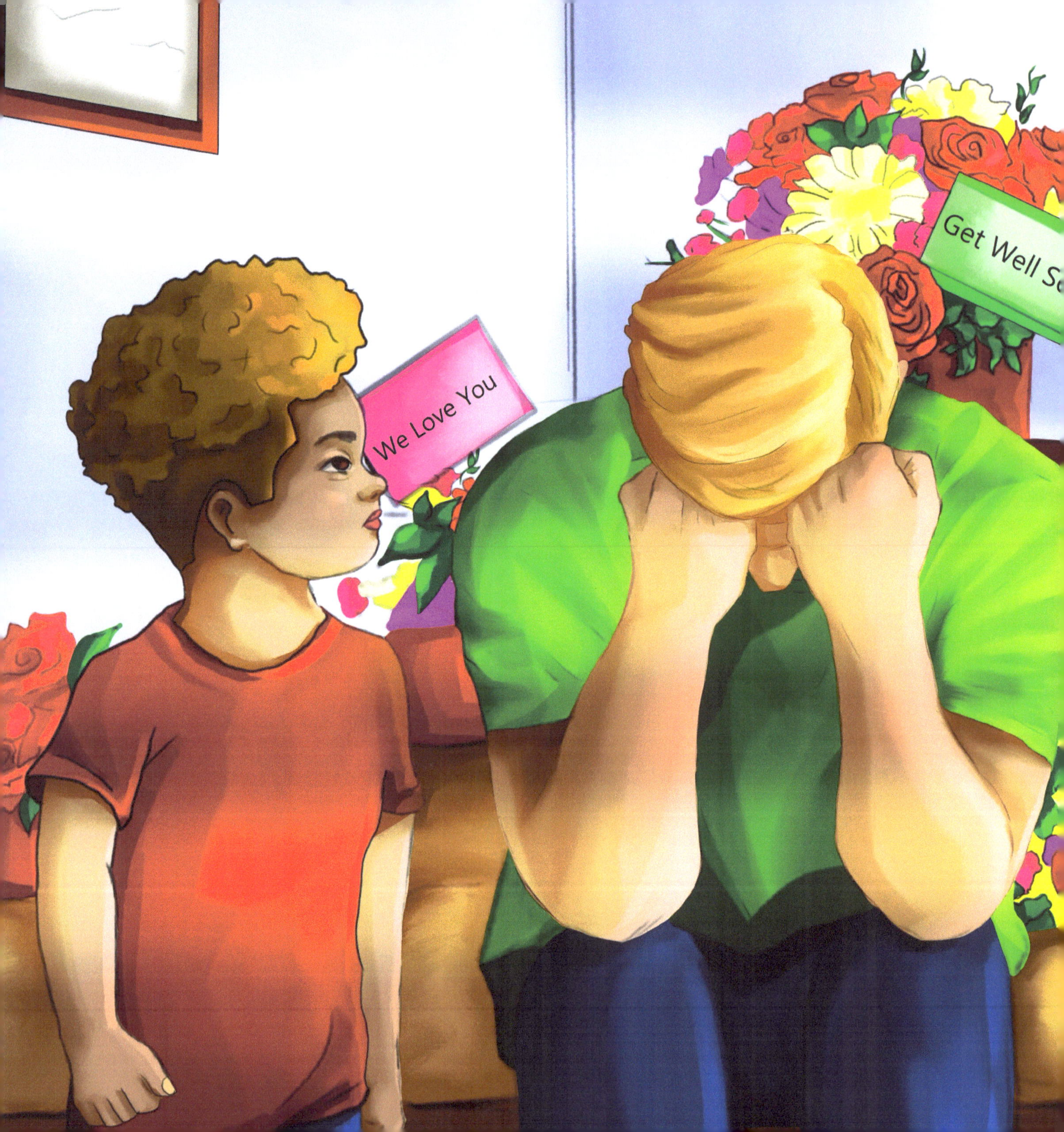

We Love You
Get Well So

Mummy cannot yet believe it
Daddy angry seems to be
I really don't understand it
What will happen next for me?

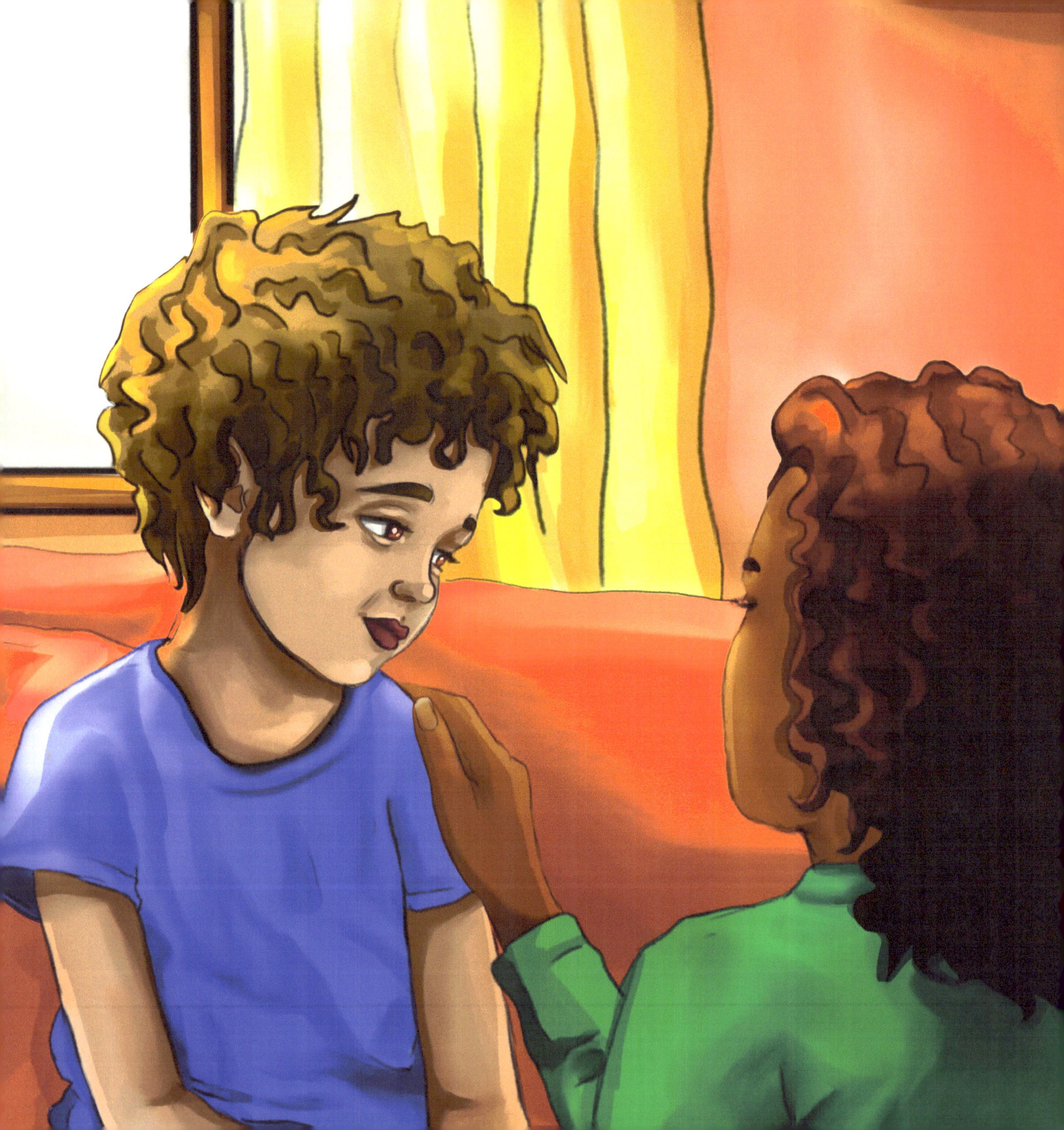

Mummy says the baby is gone
I wonder why, I feel alone
The doctors couldn't save him
There is nothing to be done

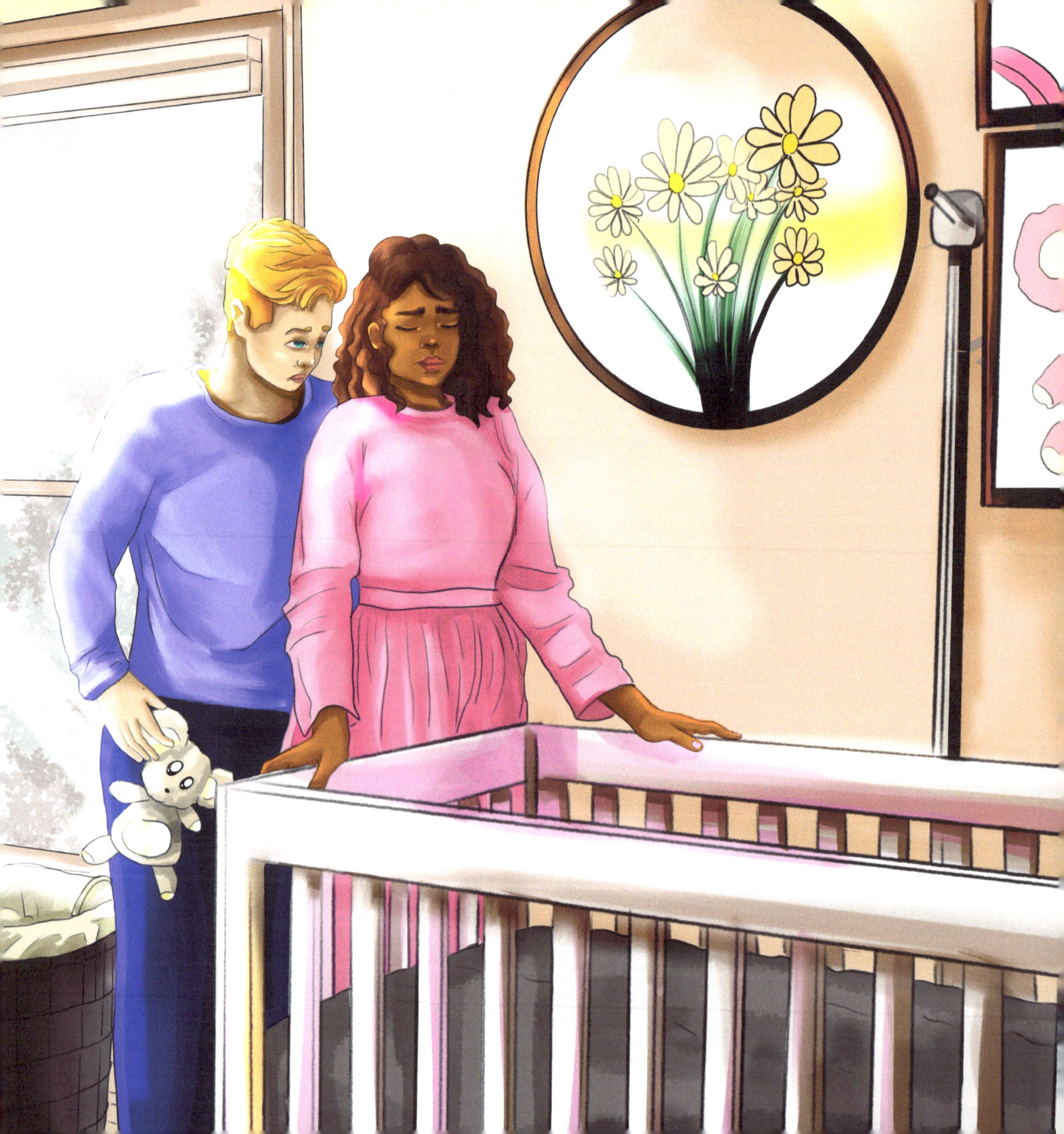

The baby is not coming home
His room is filled with emptiness
Our lives have to go on
But will the sadness ever be less?

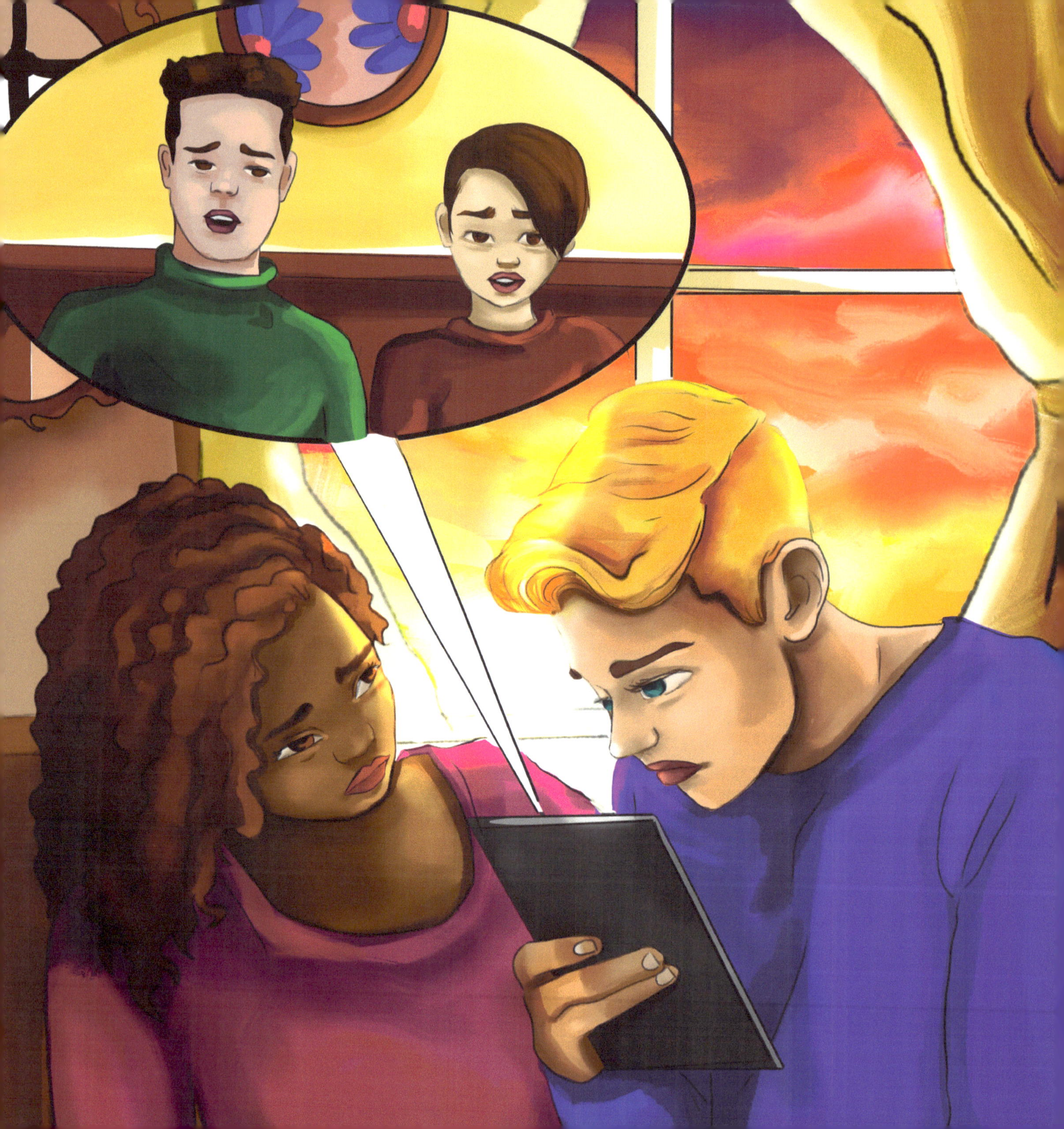

We must share with friends and family
They will feel our loss and sorrow
A grief shared is half a grief
And we begin again tomorrow

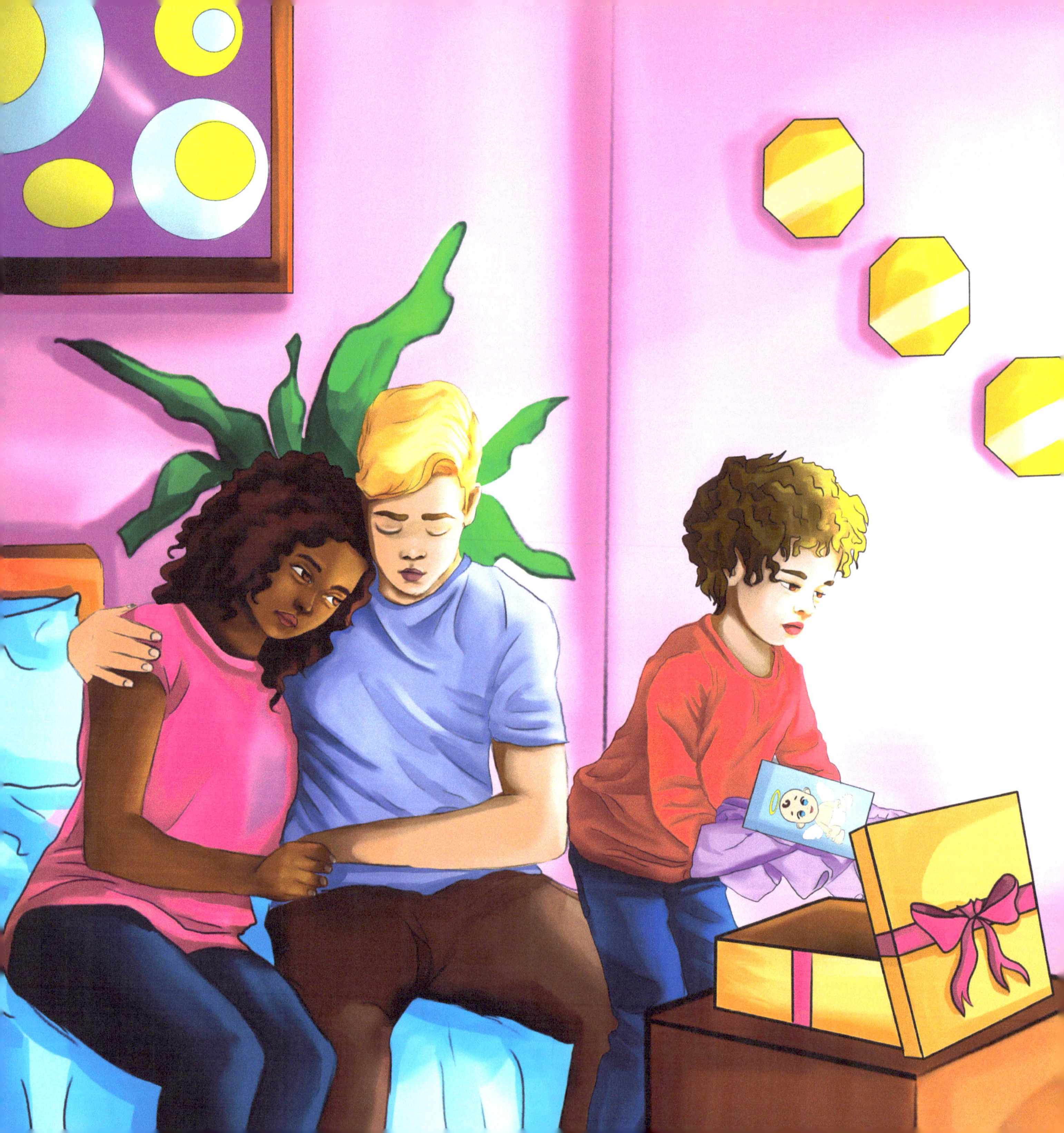

In our memories you'll be
Although you never got to live
With this keepsake box we'll remember
The part of our family you will always be

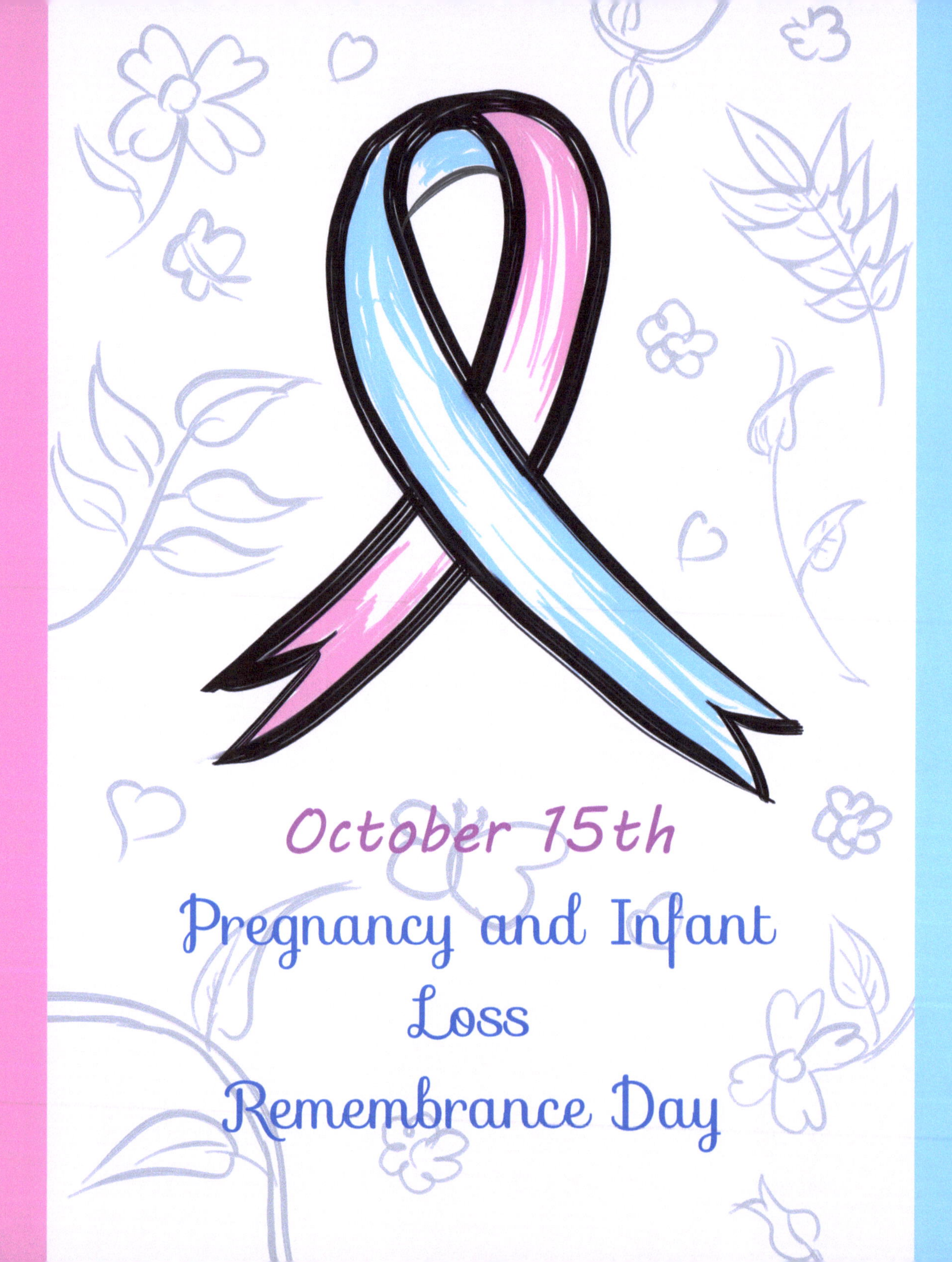

October 15th
Pregnancy and Infant
Loss
Remembrance Day